The Dark Womb Redemption 2

A guide to pregnancy, childbirth and postpartum

Abena Adu

Printed in the United States of America
First Printing, 2019
ISBN 9798322023791

Published by The Crafts Wombman

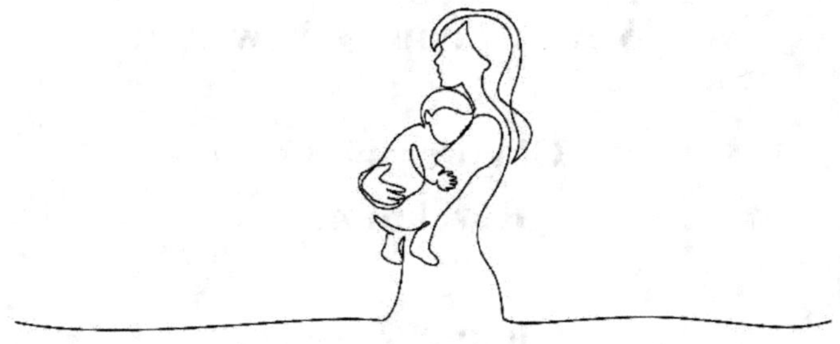

Introduction

If you want to locate an upscale, modernized hospital in America, that task won't be difficult. There are so many of them. The specialized physicians are plentiful as well. Despite all of the upgrades and technology booming in the healthcare system, the infant and maternal mortality rates among Black women are skyrocketing. There is much blame to go around. We can surely try to change the broken system that was never created with our benefit in mind. I support the action of reform; however, I would like for expectant families to do everything that they can to improve their birth experiences on their own.

The preparation must begin before conception. By getting our bodies physically and emotionally ready in advance can prevent many of the problems that arise later on. Our babies should be intentionally conceived. Then after conception, the pregnancy should be taken very seriously. As we plan for the day of birth, we must plan for the postpartum period as well.

As a doula of 15 years and womb wellness specialist of 10 years, I now see how consistent preparation makes a great difference. I am a mother and have experienced the worst and best of child birthing. I've witnessed firsthand how exercising, eating healthy, changing your mindset and being confident can improve your experience.

In this book, I am going to present to you an effective plan for you to follow so that you can have pleasant results in the prenatal, delivery and postpartum stages of your journey.

Chapter 1

A Spiritual Conception

We learned in biology class how babies are created. The sperm meet the egg; fertilization occurs creating a zygote. The zygote becomes an embryo. The embryo becomes a fetus, then grows into an infant. This is a straightforward scientific explanation. However, there is a spiritual component that I don't hear about. It's not a surprise, because conception in itself is a mystery on a deeper level. Some people may refer to it as ancestral. There are cultures who believe that we choose our parents in the spiritual realm before we are born. Some people believe in reincarnation and/or we are returned ancestors. There are so many religious and spiritual concepts when it comes to impregnation and childbearing. The unexplainable fact of conception is that something unseen becomes seen.

The Calling

There are what I call "oops babies." I am one of them. My parents did not plan to have me, but here

I am. Many "oops babies" are aborted or lost through miscarriage and stillbirths. Some "oops babies" grow up to disrupt the flow of things and change the world. Everyone has a purpose.

In my opinion, it is best to plan your conception one to two years in advance. Start by selecting a proper mate to start your family. Ask about their health status and family background. Meet their family members, friends, co-workers and spend a lot of time together to become familiar with their true personality. Examine and prepare your finances to take care of a dependent, although it can seem as though you can never ever attain enough money to take care of a child. Get your physical body in the best shape to carry and give birth to your baby. Rearrange, organize and plan your next steps in life in order to offer your child the best beginning that is possible.

Equip your physical body by addressing any health concerns that may present a challenge for you. Think about what your future income will be with the pregnancy and postpartum breaks in mind. Solidify your relationship with your partner. Discuss and come into an agreement on the decision of bringing a baby into this world.

Your child or children may appear in your dreams before they are born. You may feel a burning desire that won't go away when it's time for you to conceive, and it goes far beyond the temporary feeling of an orgasm. Watch and look for the spiritual signs. Listen to yourself. Follow your intuition.

When you both have agreed to try to conceive, plan accordingly. Familiarize yourself with your menstrual/ovulation cycle. As you answer that spiritual call, make that time special. Pray, meditate and think only good thoughts. Surround yourself in peace, keep your vibrations high and dwell in a positive atmosphere. Be intentional and do what it takes to conceive. Make love!

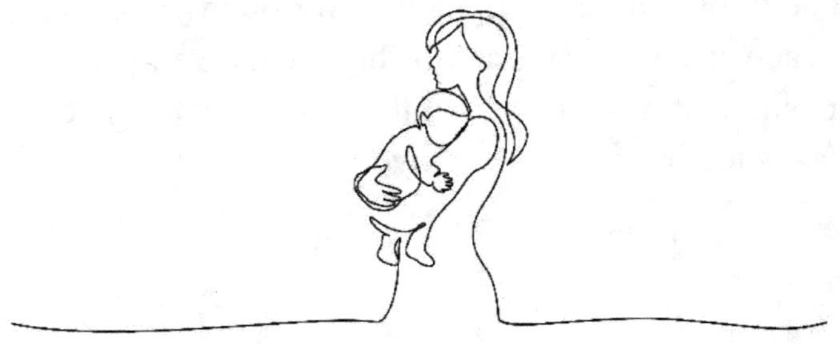

Chapter 2

Sacred Seed

It is done

You did it!

You took the pregnancy test, and the result was positive. Get ready to blossom into a new being as you grow your baby inside. Before you go around announcing the good news, sit within this new reality yourself. I recommend waiting after three months *(1st trimester)* to share with anyone other than your spouse, of course, and maybe your employer if your work duties need to be modified due to the pregnancy. In my opinion, making the decision to wait longer and maybe only tell a few people is a good decision.

Pregnancy is such a spiritual moment. Guard yourself accordingly: create your own energetic protection shield.

Determine what kind of birth you want to have, and select the people that you want to be a part of your birth team during this precious time. Consider hiring a doula, which can be one of the most important people within your support group.

DON'T BIRTH WITHOUT A DOULA

A doula is a support person who can care for you (non-medically) before, during and after your delivery. Birth or labor doulas assist you from the beginning of pregnancy to just after labor. Postpartum doulas usually start after you've returned home from delivering your baby. They will arrive at your home and help you with your requested tasks. The duties vary based on the client's needs and desires. Although a doula is like a sister, friend or aunt, she is a professional. Although there are no standard regulations, licensing or guidelines, most doulas go through training and meet certain requirements to become certified.

Please take the time and interview several doulas to determine which one that you want to help you during such a vulnerable time.

Doulas literally save lives. They are knowledgeable to know the signs and warnings of illnesses and emergencies. They can direct you to the proper physicians and medical facilities. You only spend a short amount of time with your doctor or midwife, but most likely you will have 24-hour access to your doula.

Some may think that a doula will interfere or get in the way of the family during the labor, but an experienced and trained doula knows her place. They are there to support, not be a nuisance. Doulas support the birthing family also, not just the birthing mother.

Doulas may or may not:

- Help you to locate a doctor or midwife
- Attend prenatal appointments with you
- Offer nutritional advice
- Create an exercise plan for you
- Attend your birth the entire time that you are in active labor
- Help you with birthing positions and breathing techniques while in labor
- Help you with breastfeeding
- Help you with postpartum care
- Cook and/or deliver meals to you
- Help you with your newborn
- Help with house cleaning or running errands

The price of a doula will vary based on the education, experience and level of service that will be provided. It could cost a few hundred or thousands of dollars. There should be a signed agreement *(contract),* between you and the doula that clearly entails what the doula will do and the total balance due.

Birth Team

Diligently set aside the time to select the members of your birth team, birth location and decide which type of birth that you are planning on having.

Your birth team may or may not include:

- Spouse and/or baby's other parent
- Midwife or OB/GYN
- Doula
- Family Member
- Friend
- Chiropractor
- Massage Therapist

Carefully research the background of each potential birth team member. Check to see if there are any complaints on the medical board, health department and/or licensing websites. Search for any listed client reviews. Ask other people who may be familiar with them about their reputation.

Be sure to visit hospitals and birth centers in advance to select the best place to birth. Write down the questions that you want to ask before you arrive. Listen to your intuition, it is usually heightened and accurate while pregnant. Remember it is okay to change your mind about any decision that you may have previously made.

Type of Birth

<u>Freebirth</u> — Mother receives no medical prenatal or postpartum care. There is no medical supervision at birth.

<u>Unassisted Birth</u> — Mother may receive medical prenatal and/or postpartum care, but there is no medical supervision at birth.

<u>Home Birth</u> — Mother receives medical supervision by a midwife at birth. Prenatal and postpartum care is provided by a midwife at the mother's home or birthing center.

<u>Hospital Birth</u> — Prenatal and postpartum care is provided by an OB/GYN. Birth takes place in a hospital.

<u>Cesarean</u> — Surgical procedure performed to deliver the baby.

Water Birth — Delivery of baby in water, usually in a birth pool or bathtub. Medical supervision may or may not be present during delivery.

Lotus Birth — After delivery of the baby, the infant's umbilical cord is still attached to the placenta, until it naturally separates on its own.

Nutrition

Eating and drinking in a healthy manner is vital when you are pregnant. At this precious stage, weight loss diets are not safe. Don't worry about your weight gain; just focus on supplying your body with a variety of healthy food. The cells that your baby is made of are dependent on what you put in your body.

Consider your health status. You may be deficient in certain vitamins and minerals. If you decide to take prenatal vitamins, find the best supplements that will absorb in the body well. Read the label ingredients and research anything that may be unknown to you.

Don't ever skip breakfast. Pregnancy is not the time to go on a weight loss diet. Be very conscious of what you eat. Go for a wide range of colorful foods that include lots of fresh fruits, vegetables, grains and legumes. Limit the consumption of heavily processed foods. Don't stress yourself about healthy eating; just have the best of what's available to you.

Keep yourself well hydrated. I've had many pregnant women tell me that they don't want to drink so much, because it causes them to urinate too often. No matter how inconvenient it is, you need to drink healthy beverages. Be sure to incorporate smoothies and tea to your list of drinks, but water should be your favorite drink. Your baby is living in water. Your body is made of mostly water. Dehydration can cause health problems leading to pregnancy complications.

In my opinion, red raspberry leaf is good for pregnancy because it strengthens and tones the uterus for the growing baby. Chamomile may be good for stress relief, relaxation and insomnia. Ginger can help eliminate nausea. Sea moss can provide the body with essential vitamins and minerals. Nettle is an excellent source of iron. *Get an approval from your physician before taking any herbs and/or supplements.*

<u>Constipation</u>
Pregnant women may complain about passing stools at some point during their pregnancy. This is usually an easy fix. Eat meals with a high fiber

content, which could include beans, raw or lightly cooked vegetables and fresh fruits. Drinking water and exercising can relieve constipation.

Rest

During the 1st trimester, although you may not be showing that baby bump yet, severe fatigue is common. Because of a growing fetus, your organs are making way for the baby, and it can feel physically overwhelming. When you are tired, please sleep. Don't feel guilty about it. Those extra hours of shut eye are needed.

When the 2nd trimester arrives, you may feel a burst of energy. Enjoy it because the fatigue will return. This may be the time to take that trip and benefit from the ability to be active without feeling sluggish.

Toward the end of the 3rd trimester, exhaustion returns. The body is still expanding. Signs of anxiety may also arise. Whenever you can, sleep. Exercise should still be practiced, but be sure to take breaks in between and stay hydrated by drinking water.

Movement

Exercise is necessary. The benefits are abundant. Movement is mandatory and it is essential to maintain good health. Doing regular cardio, aerobics or pilates can help eliminate anxiety. Getting the blood flowing relieves the body of stress and can improve your mood.

One study found significant improvement in the fatigue levels of expecting women who walked just 30 minutes four times a week.

The first and third trimesters can be very tiring. Be gentle with yourself in the beginning of your pregnancy. As long as you're not put on bed rest, push through and exercise during your last trimester. It will help you have a smoother labor and faster postpartum recovery.
Consult your physician for approval before starting any exercise regimen.

As you exercise, realize that you are improving your muscle tone, bone health, cell development, blood volume and organ capacity. All of this will benefit you and your baby.
Exercise is supposed to be a way of life: it's not about weight loss or improving your physical look. It's about strengthening your body for childbirth

and having a speedy postpartum recovery. Movement increases energy levels. It helps with insomnia. Your risk of complications while pregnant, during labor, and postpartum are greatly decreased. Staying physically active may benefit not only pregnancy and labor, but also postpartum healing.

Remain consistent with moving your body, but never overexert yourself. Take breaks anytime that you feel like it. If you feel tired or weak, stop immediately. Drink sips of water just before, during and after your workout. Wait at least one hour after eating before beginning any exercise routine. Wear comfortable clothing, socks and shoes. Barefoot for certain exercises can be better. Keep a clean hand towel for sweating that may occur.

Walking is an underrated exercise. To some it takes very little effort and for others it can be a great challenge. Be grateful for the ability to walk. Walking can reduce pregnancy complications, decreasing the risk of gestational diabetes and preeclampsia. It keeps your back muscles strong and supports your growing belly, while also eliminating stiffness. Keep walking to reduce pain and prevent constipation. Because you are working out the abdominal muscles, it can help you have the strength to push your baby out.

Swimming is one of the best exercises for pregnancy. It works out the entire body and is gentle on the joints. It strengthens underworked muscles. It's comfortable during pregnancy and its low impact. It also has mood-boosting benefits. It improves blood flow to the brain. Swimming is also fun.

Stretching is a must. It decreases the risk of prenatal depression, improves sleep, decreases back pain and nausea. It improves stamina, calms the nervous system, improves flexibility/balance while reducing mood swings. It can help you to center yourself, become grounded and confident.

- To help with <u>fluid retention</u> and <u>ankle swelling</u>, put legs up on the wall making an L shape. The pressure gets diverted in that position and can create balance.

- To strengthen and maintain flexibility in the <u>lower back</u> and <u>abdomen</u>, do the cow and cat pose. Get on your hands and knees, with hands and knees shoulder width apart. Round, hump your back, then relax your back, allowing it to sink down.

<u>**Squatting**</u> strengthens pelvic floor muscles and prevents back and pelvic pain. It is excellent in preparing the body for labor. It strengthens your legs, and strong legs give you more endurance in your birthing positions. Squats can help a baby descend deeper down into the pelvis.

Only go as far down you can. It should be comfortable; don't strain, force or overextend yourself. Use a pillow to rest your bottom on as support. Bend down resting on pillows, legs open, back straight, hands in prayer position.

Recommended pregnancy exercise routine

1st trimester
WALK daily — 20 minutes,
STRETCH daily — 20 minutes,
SQUATS — 20 count

2nd trimester
WALK daily — 30 minutes,
STRETCH daily — 30 minutes,
SWIM once per week — 30 minutes,
SQUATS — 30 count

3rd trimester
WALK daily — 45 minutes,
STRETCH daily — 30 minutes,
SWIM twice per week — 30 minutes,
SQUATS — 40 count

Yoga Ball

The yoga ball, also known as a *"fitness ball"* or *"birthing ball,"* is a great investment during pregnancy. It's proven to be a great benefit when used in prenatal exercise, stretching and during labor. This useful prop is a gift that keeps on giving. It can be used at any stage in life, from pregnancy to beyond postpartum. Consider using a yoga ball. Stretching with it can prevent injury. Exercising with it is a great way to relieve back pressure and stiffness.

Yoga balls are larger for comfort and have an anti-slip finish. They come in different sizes. You should be able to sit on it comfortably with your feet flat on the floor. Choose the ball size according to your height. The manufacturers have recommendations on the packaging to help you decide which size is a right fit for you. Be sure to get the right size or else it would be counter-productive, causing knee and back pain.

<u>**Ways to use a yoga ball**</u>

Simply sit on the ball instead of using a chair. Allow your body to make circles, figure 8's, rock back and forth. Put your hands on your hips and roll your waist. Gently sway from side to side. Get creative with the motion; it all helps the abdominal and back muscles get stimulated. It can also improve posture and increase blood flow to all the muscles around the pelvic region.

Lean your chest on the yoga ball while on your knees. Let the arms hang alongside. This can relieve neck and back pain.

Elevate your legs and rest both calves on top of the ball, while you lie down on your back. Move your waist in a circular motion, move your legs from side to side on the ball. This movement can improve circulation.

Bouncing and sitting upright on the yoga ball can also encourage your baby to get into a great laboring position. Try using the yoga ball to turn a breech or transverse positioned baby. It may also change a baby from a posterior position to an anterior position, which may also alleviate back pain.

I recommend using the yoga ball while in labor. It can decrease pelvic pressure and may even shorten labor. After delivery, it can become your new seat because of the comfort it gives. After postpartum healing, it can also be used to help you get in shape and reach your fitness goals.

Clean your ball with a towel, water and mild soap. If you're laboring on it without any underwear, place a clean towel or chuck pad on top of it.

Sexual Intercourse during pregnancy

Sexual intimacy is a good thing. If you are advised to abstain for safety reasons, please follow your medical instructions.

Sexual activity is a great way for you to bond with your partner. It improves the mood and releases stress. Being active in that way can create an easier labor experience because the uterus is getting stronger. It may be easier to handle contractions/surges and quicken labor by loosening up the pelvic muscles. Intercourse releases stagnant energy in the womb and lowers blood pressure. Orgasms create contractions/surges and can be a natural labor inducer. Avoid if you don't desire that type of intimacy; don't feel pressured to go against your innate feelings. Refrain from it, if it is painful and also if there's an infection in that area and/or bleeding/spotting.

Medical technology during pregnancy

In this modern society, medical technology is often used at prenatal doctor visits. It is convenient for use by the medical staff but can also be costly for the patient. Medical technologies, such as fetal heart monitoring and ultrasounds, may be risky. Be certain to research and question all medical technologies being used on you while you are pregnant and also during labor. Sometimes certain testing and getting your blood withdrawn excessively can be refused. Well, actually you can refuse any medical treatment.

Consent

When you give someone permission or come into an agreement to do something, you are giving consent. Be mindful of people (strangers, family members, medical staff, etc.) touching you without your consent. The prenatal stage is such a delicate one, you may feel more sensitive. Pregnant women are beautiful and magnetizing. Some people can't help themselves and will touch you, specifically your belly without asking or considering your feelings. Don't feel obligated to let everyone touch you. It's quite all right to shield yourself with some sort of physical covering. You can simply say, "I don't want to be touched."

Ultrasounds

This medical imaging test utilizes high frequency sound waves to create images of soft tissue inside of your body. The technician should be well trained and experienced in performing this test. Prolonged use can create heat in the body and the long-term risks may be unknown. In my opinion, it may be best to avoid ultrasounds within the 1st trimester and limit them later on in the pregnancy.

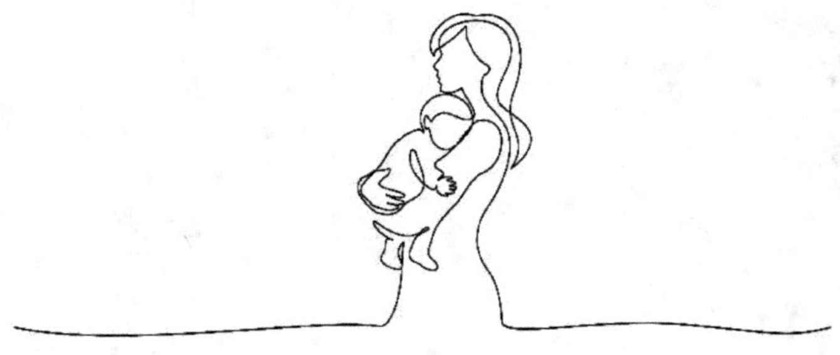

Chapter 3

Word ~ Sound ~ Power

BONDING

Although you can't hold your baby in your arms yet or physically see them (besides through ultrasounds), you can still form a strong bond with your baby through sound. Babies can hear in utero. The baby is constantly listening to the rhythm of your heartbeat. Sing a song to soothe your baby. If you repeat the same song regularly, your baby will even remember the song once they are born.

Place your hands on your belly. Send positive energy to your baby. From your hands, through your belly to the baby. Speak great words. When you're not speaking, send them telepathic messages.

I believe that when you are in tune with your baby in utero, you are simultaneously in tune with yourself, therefore decreasing the chances of pregnancy and labor complications.

Cut out the mental chatter, and limit your screen time television and useless conversations.

Bonding will solidify a lifelong shatterproof relationship.

How to write a Birth Plan

A birth plan is your birth vision written down on paper. Make a few copies and give them to the people on your birth team who will be assisting you during your delivery. Having a birth plan helps your supporting people adhere to your wishes, without having to ask you while you are in labor. Unexpected events may occur, so it would be a good idea to also include plan B options. Here are some questions that you may want to answer and list on your birth plan.

- Who would you like to be with you during your birth?
- Create your playlist. What type of music would you prefer?
- Are there any tools that you desire? Examples: fan, massager, yoga ball, etc.
- Are there any colors that make you feel calm? Would you like a personal theme?

- Do you like certain scents? What type of essential oils, incense, candles?
- Do you prefer to have pain medication, epidural or none at all?
- Would you like delayed cord clamping?
- Do you want your baby to receive shots?
- Would you like for your newborn to receive eye ointment?
- Would you like to delay your newborn's first bath?

Stress Management

Stress is the pressure and/or reaction to something seen as a threat, challenge or barrier. We all experience stress in life. Relaxing is the key to countering it all. When the muscles are relaxed, everything in the body can function without resistance.

Be mindful of your stress levels while pregnant. Your baby can feel every emotion you feel, so guard your heart and spirit. Stay away from negative people and situations as much as possible. Limit your time, being in the presence of negativity. Try your best to feel good and focus on positivity. It all starts in your mind, so control your thoughts. Create a habit of having only happy thoughts. Write in your ***Pregnancy Journal***.

Birth Language

Replace the word "contractions" with surges, blossoming, opening, preparing the uterus or riding the wave.

Replace the word "pain" with pressure, intensity, or uncomfortable.

Once you and your birth team switch out these two words, this change can create a more positive atmosphere surrounding your birth and shift things during your delivery.

Positive self-talk can change your thoughts, then your reality. Manifestation is real. Speaking affirmations can help build up your confidence, activate muscles and increase your energy. Develop a habit of speaking affirmations, especially when you may be feeling down.

PREGNANCY AFFIRMATIONS

These affirmations are positive statements designed for personal encouragement, relaxation, eliminating anxiety and fears. My intent on sharing them is that you will have a pleasant pregnancy and birth experience.

Place your hands on your belly. Slow down your breathing, focus on inhaling and exhaling for a few minutes. Then began to speak these affirmations below.

I AM SO HAPPY TO BE EXPECTING

I WELCOME AN AMAZING PREGNANCY JOURNEY

I HONOR MY BODY

I AM GRATEFUL TO BE FERTILE

I LOVE MYSELF AND MY BABY

I AM REGENERATING

I RESPECT THIS PREGNANCY

I FEEL GREAT ABOUT REPRODUCING MYSELF

I AM FRUITFUL

I AM FLEXIBLE

I LIKE BEING PREGNANT

I ENJOY THE SPECIAL TREATMENT

I CHOSE LIFE

LIFE CHOSE ME

I AM GRATEFUL THAT WE CHOSE EACH
OTHER

MY WOMB IS A SAFE SPACE

I AM SURROUNDED BY SO MUCH
SUPPORT

HELP IS ALL AROUND ME

I TRUST THIS PROCESS

I NOURISH MYSELF & MY BABY

I AM ADAPTING WELL TO THE CHANGES
GOING ON WITHIN MY BODY

I FEEL COMFORTABLE

I AM CARRYING MY BABY WELL

WE ARE PROTECTED

I AM GRATEFUL TO HAVE THIS
EXPERIENCE

THIS PREGNANCY IS A BREEZE

I ENJOY MOVING AND STAYING IN SHAPE

I LISTEN TO MY BODY

I REST EASY WHEN I'M SLEEPING

I AM AT PEACE

I AM ENJOYING THIS PREGNANCY

EVERYTHING THAT I DESIRE I RECEIVE

MY BELLY IS FULL OF EXCELLENCE

MY BELLY IS FULL OF PERFECTION
I AM PREPARING TO BIRTH BRILLIANCE

MY SUPERPOWERS ARE INCREASING

I HAVE LIGHT SHINING INSIDE OF ME
MY BODY KNOWS EXACTLY WHAT IT IS
DOING

I AM THANKFUL FOR A HEALTHY
PREGNANCY

I TOTALLY LOVE MY BODY

I AM WISE

I AM CONFIDENT

MY BODY IS HEALTHY AND ADJUSTING
WELL

I BREATHE EASILY

MY HEALTH CONTINUES TO IMPROVE

I AM CAPABLE OF HAVING A
SUCCESSFUL BIRTH

I WILL BE A GOOD MOTHER

HOW I FEEL MATTERS

I AM GRATEFUL FOR MY ABILITY TO
CARRY LIFE

I AM HEALTHY AND HAPPY RIGHT NOW

I SEND MY BABY LOVING THOUGHTS

I HAVE EVERYTHING THAT IT TAKES TO GIVE BIRTH

I WILL BIRTH AT THE RIGHT TIME

THERE IS NO RUSH

I BREATHE SLOWLY AND CALMLY

MY BABY WILL COME OUT SO EASY

I LOOK FORWARD TO MY BABY'S BIRTH

I AM EXCITED TO DELIVER

THIS BIRTH WILL BE PERFECT

PREGNANCY MEDITATION

Go to a place where you can retreat from the world. It should be a quiet place, then turn on some meditation or reiki music. Get into a comfortable position. It may be sitting or lying down.

*Now breathe. Inhale and exhale slowly.
Intentionally release the tension in every part of
your body. From the top of your head to the soles
of your feet. Relax your eyebrows, neck, fingers,
back, ankles, etc. Close your eyes and continue
breathing slowly.*

*Imagine yourself moving through a rainforest.
You could be floating, walking or even flying. This
is your moment, visualize yourself in the way that
you want to move.*

*The weather is perfect. You walk down a pathway
that leads you to water. You are now standing in a
warm waterfall. Feel the water gently massaging
your body. Enjoy the natural shower. Feel the
refreshment. Be thankful for the beauty and
freedom around you.
Envision yourself having a calm, controlled birth,
birthing in the position that you want to give birth
in. You have the power to create your own reality.
You are birthing without fear. Everything is
flowing well, just as you'd like it to.*

*Feel the safety of your comfortable environment.
There is no rush. Just surrender to the process.
Imagine your baby sliding out of your body. You
are congratulated by those around you.*

You look at your baby snuggled in your arms. Welcome the feeling of joy.

Take some long deep breaths, then when you are ready, open your eyes.

POSTPARTUM PLAN

There is so much emphasis on the actual day of birth, the postpartum period is often overlooked. This portion of time deserves much planning and preparation, too.

List the answers to these questions on your postpartum plan.

- Who will provide food for you?
- Who will handle the household duties, such as laundry, housecleaning, etc.?
- Who will maintain your hair for you?
- Who will take care of your other children or pets?
- When will you return to work?
- Who will care for your newborn when you are not able to do so?
- Will you have a breast pumping schedule?

- When will you make time for yourself to be pampered?
- Are you going to do vaginal steams?
- Are you going to belly bind?

Chapter 4

Revelation

While you are in gestation and years afterward, the level of vulnerability cannot be explained or determined. As strong and knowledgeable as you may be, you are fragile like a glass cup. A glass cup is important and useful, durable and able to hold liquid and solid contents. Then within a quick second, by a forceful strike, it can be shattered into pieces and unable to hold anything. This metaphor is related to pregnancy, birthing and post-delivery.

Medical Interventions

A medical intervention is when a person from the medical staff interferes with a normal or natural process. It may or may not be necessary. Please question everything. Do your own research and trust your gut. Here are some medical interventions related to labor and delivery.

- Induction (start labor)
- Artificial Rupture of Membranes (breaking your waters)

- Episiotomy (cut made between the vagina and anus)
- Cesarean (cut in abdomen and uterus to remove infant)

As much as you have planned and prepared for an outcome, please understand that there could be a change in your birth plans due to complications. It's important to consider the risks and benefits to you and your baby if having an intervention. It is also important to consider any risks associated with declining or consenting to an intervention.

DELAYED CORD CLAMPING

The medical establishments have now recognized that delaying the cord clamping can be highly beneficial for the newborn. It can be done after a vaginal or C-section delivery.

Delaying the cord clamping in full-term infants may include decreased risk of anemia, better establishment of red blood volume, lower incidence of hemorrhage in baby's brain and more.

The amount of time to wait varies. Some medical professionals wait 30 seconds to 5 minutes. In my opinion, if there is no medical emergency to deviate from delayed cord clamping, I would suggest waiting until the cord stops pulsating and it turns white.

PLACENTA

There is so much information now available about the placenta. It grows in the pregnant belly alongside the baby. The placenta provides nourishment to the fetus. It attaches to the uterus and is also connected to the umbilical cord.

The remarkable placenta organ is a rich source of stem cells with immense potential for medical advancement.

Some mothers are choosing to ingest their babies' placenta in capsule form to receive the nutritional and emotional healing benefits. After delivery, the placenta is washed and kept cool until the encapsulation process. It is cleansed again, steamed, dried, then ground into a fine powder before filling into capsules.

Some practitioners of <u>placenta encapsulation</u> believe that it offers the mom an increased milk production, a reduction in postpartum depression and faster healing process.

Since the placenta is filled with nutrients, some families may choose to bury it into the earth. It may be tossed in a river or lake, at the root of a tree or in their personal garden.

The practice of keeping the placenta attached to the umbilical cord until it naturally dries and falls off is called a "lotus birth." Proponents of lotus birth believe it may increase hemoglobin levels and decrease the need for blood transfusion. They also claim that it is a less-invasive transition for the baby as they enter the world from the womb, a spiritual way to honor the life shared between the baby and placenta.

How to do a lotus birth

Materials

Large bowl, Strainer, Towel, Herbs (lavender, rose, rosemary), Sea Salt, 100% Pure Essential Oils (lavender, cedarwood, tea tree), Bag or container

Instructions

- Wash off placenta with strainer underneath, pat dry with a clean towel
- Place placenta inside bag or leak free container
- Rub with herbs, cover with sea salt
- Add several drops of essential oils to it

Breastfeeding

Breastfeeding will be challenging at first. Your nipples will become supple as you have a hungry newborn suckling milk out of them. Its miraculous force can be draining, but it is all worth it. Breastfeeding your baby is the best way to feed your baby. Not only is the baby getting the best nourishment for optimal health, but the uterus is also benefiting from it as well. While you breastfeed, your uterus contracts. It tones up and may prevent you from diseases in that area.

Breastfeeding is also referred to as "nursing." You are caring for your baby in a special way when you breastfeed. If you have made the choice to breastfeed, please stick to it. You can overcome the challenges; just be consistent. It does get greater later. The benefits outweigh a decision to quit.

I encourage nursing your baby if it is possible, but if you are having problems, please seek help. A doula and/or lactation consultant can provide assistance. There are also milk banks available that offer donor milk. Ask around for breast milk from a healthy nursing mother who is still lactating and/or has stored frozen breast milk. Offer her something in return to show your appreciation because pumping breast milk is work.

I have over eight years of breastfeeding experience combined. Although there were challenging times, I never gave up. I know what it's like to have no support, mastitis, fatigue, etc. I knew that my breast milk was better than any infant formula. Through all the ups and downs, I remained consistent in my choice, and I have no regrets. All of my children are healthy and intelligent. I do believe that exclusively (without formula) and extensively (breastfeeding past age 1) nursing them, helped with that.

VULNERABLE ACKNOWLEDGMENT

During this fragile time, you will need more help than you realize. Don't feel ashamed to ask, and own no feelings of guilt when accepting the invitation of help. The process of bringing life into this world is no small feat. It takes a toll on your physical body and mental space. It's quite normal to have a variety of emotions throughout the day. Everyday won't be easy and everyday won't be hard.

VICTORY IS YOURS

Having a baby is life changing. You may feel
powerful at one minute, then hopeless the next.
Don't give in to the sadness. Every step is a phase.
Every phase may present new challenges. Rise
above all of the negative emotions and know that
"This too shall pass."

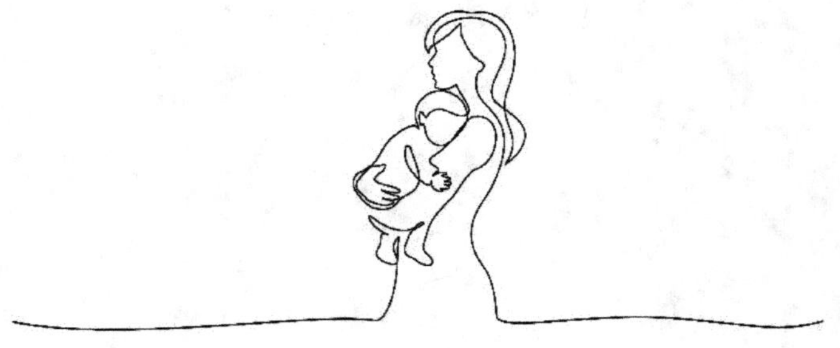

Chapter 5

Mama's Re-Birth

"When a mother is giving birth to her baby, she is also giving birth to herself."

CHILDBIRTH AFFIRMATIONS

Once you start the process of birthing your baby, speak these affirmations. Your support person may also read them to you as well.

GIVE THANKS FOR LIFE

THIS IS DIVINE TIME

MY BODY IS PREPARING TO BRING MY BABY HERE

I BREATHE MY BABY DOWN AND OUTSIDE MY BODY

I CAN DO THIS

I FEEL LOVE ALL AROUND ME

**THIS BIRTH IS MAGICAL
I WELCOME THIS PROCESS**

TODAY IS THE BEST DAY OF MY LIFE

EVERYTHING IS ALIGNED

I AM RIDING THE WAVE

I AM FLEXIBLE

I FEEL CALM

MY MIND IS AT PEACE

I RESPECT BIRTH

**EVERY MOMENT I GET CLOSER TO
SEEING MY BABY**

MY BODY IS WISE

I TRUST THIS PROCESS

EVERYTHING IS FLOWING WELL

I ACCEPT BIRTH

THIS IS NORMAL

THIS IS NATURAL

**I HAVE BEEN CHOSEN TO DO WHAT SO
MANY HAVE DONE BEFORE ME**

I AM ABLE TO DELIVER

I AM PREPARED TO BIRTH

I AM PREPARED FOR MY BABY

I AM HAVING A SUCCESSFUL DELIVERY

I SAY YES TO BIRTH

**MY BABY IS COMING INTO THIS WORLD
SAFELY & QUICKLY**

**I AM LOOKING FORWARD TO
BREASTFEEDING EASILY**

**MY BODY IS MAKING AN ABUNDANT
SUPPLY OF MILK**

EVERYTHING IS WELL & GOOD

MY ORGANS ARE HEALTHY

**MY BABY IS FINE
MY BACK IS RELIEVED**

I SURRENDER TO BIRTH

I SOFTEN, I OPEN

I AM DOING A GOOD JOB

I AM SECURE IN THIS MOMENT

I LET GO

I SURRENDER TO PROCESS OF BIRTH

I PROGRESS WITH EACH SURGE

**IN MY ARMS IS WHERE MY BABY WILL
BE**

I AM READY TO OPEN THE GATEWAY

WE ARE PROTECTED

WE CAN DO THIS

I GIVE INTO THIS EXPERIENCE

I FEEL MY MUSCLES RELAXING

I AM STRONG & SO IS MY BABY
THIS IS A POSITIVE EXPERIENCE

I AM CONFIDENT

I AM A WOMAN

MY BODY WAS DESIGNED TO GIVE BIRTH

MY UTERUS WILL RELEASE WITH EASE

MY MIND IS AT PEACE

I ALLOW RADIANT ENERGY TO FLOW
THROUGH ME

MY BODY KNOWS EXACTLY WHAT TO DO

MY BABY KNOWS EXACTLY WHAT TO DO

WE ARE IN HARMONY

I AM READY TO HOLD MY BABY

VERY SOON, I WILL SEE MY BABY'S FACE

I TOTALLY LOVE MY BODY

I AM STRONG ENOUGH TO BIRTH

I BREATHE EASILY

I AM CAPABLE OF HAVING
A SUCCESSFUL BIRTH

I WILL BE A GOOD MOTHER

HOW I FEEL MATTERS

I AM HEALTHY AND HAPPY RIGHT NOW

I AM PATIENT

I HAVE EVERYTHING THAT IT TAKES TO
GIVE BIRTH

I WILL BIRTH AT THE RIGHT TIME

THERE IS NO RUSH

I BREATHE SLOWLY AND CALMLY

I WILL EASE THROUGH THIS PROCESS

I AM EXCITED TO DELIVER

THIS BIRTH IS PERFECT

I CHOSE LIFE

LIFE CHOSE ME

I AM GRATEFUL THAT WE CHOSE EACH OTHER

I AM SURROUNDED BY SO MUCH SUPPORT

HELP IS ALL AROUND ME

I TRUST THIS PROCESS

I FEEL COMFORTABLE

I AM GRATEFUL TO HAVE THIS EXPERIENCE

EVERYTHING THAT I DESIRE I RECEIVE

MY BELLY IS FULL OF EXCELLENCE

I AM BIRTHING GREATNESS

MY SUPERPOWERS ARE INCREASING

MY BODY KNOWS EXACTLY WHAT IT IS DOING

(Insert baby's name) _______________________

WILL SOON BE HERE

WE ARE WAITING FOR YOU

WE ARE READY FOR YOU

IMMEDIATELY AFTER BIRTH

Your voice should be the first voice that your baby hears. Start to speak to your baby; say whatever you want to say.

The first 24 hours of your newborn's life is important and even more so within the first hour of life, which is referred to as "the golden hour." Don't feel pressured to have around you during this time people whom you are uncomfortable with. This may include medical staff, family members, and/or friends. You can request that alone time with your baby and/or spouse only. You can't re-do this precious time. Make your desires known.

POSTPARTUM CARE TIPS

- Practice slow walking.
- Use an elevator or escalator whenever it is possible.
- Keep your legs closed often *(for vaginal birth)*.
- Don't be afraid to ask for help.
- Eat lots of soups and salads. Drink lots of smoothies.
- Drink water and herbal teas to remain hydrated.
- Sit on a yoga ball for a few minutes at a time throughout the day.
- Sleep/rest often.

Postpartum Self-Care Routine (25 minutes)

Disclaimer: Consult your physician for approval before implementing any of these exercises in your routine. Do not do any physical movement exercises if you are in pain or need to rest.

- 5 minutes — Walk slowly
- 5 minutes — Practice yoga poses found in the book ***The Dark Womb Redemption***.
- 5 minutes — Speak affirmations found in the book ***The Dark Womb Redemption***.
- 5 minutes — Sit comfortably and massage breasts and belly with your desired natural oil.
- 5 minutes — Lie down flat, with legs outstretched alongside the body, legs extended, palms facing the floor. Practice slow deep breathing.

Don't worry yourself with dieting and weight loss soon after birth. Just make sure that you are eating plenty of healthy foods and beverages.

Remember, although you may feel energized and ready to go after birth, you still need to go slow and allow your insides to heal.

Stay away from negative people and stressful situations.

Herbal Womb/Vaginal Steam Treatment

Disclaimer: Consult your physician for the approval of any herbal or steam use.

This ancient herbal genital treatment is exceptionally beneficial after childbirth. It can repair the perineum muscles and help release any retained placenta fragments. Sitting or squatting over the medicinal herbs may tighten the vaginal walls, tone the reproductive organs, balance the hormones, relieve stress, eliminate any pain/discomfort, nourish vaginal tissues, improve immunity, alleviate insomnia, release excess vaginal discharge, clear emotional blockages, relax mind/body/spirit, increase blood circulation and detox the entire body by producing regular bowel movements and sweat. This treatment may alleviate the symptoms associated with childbirth, tears, episiotomies, hemorrhoids, birth trauma, etc.

Use herbs from the list in the book ***The Dark Womb Redemption***.

Many women of various cultures outside of America practice vaginal steaming regularly for

cleansing, toning and strengthening. This tradition
is common for Africans, Asians, Caribbeans,
African Americans in the South and South
Americans.

Vaginal Steam Preparation

Drink plenty of water and herbal tea one week in advance.

<u>Materials/Equipment</u>

Metal Bowl & Pot (3 Quarts Size)
2 Quarts of Water
Toilet Seat
Womb Herbs
Large Towel
Small Pillow

<u>Instructions</u>

- Be sure that you will be undisturbed for a while. Play relaxing meditation music. Turn off or dim the lights. Light some candles to create an ambiance.

- Boil 2 quarts of filtered water

- Add 1 ounce of herbs to the metal bowl, then pour the boiling hot water onto the herbs.

- Place the metal bowl with herbs and water inside of the toilet, on top of the water that is in the toilet, then close the toilet seat lid down.

- Wait until the water has cooled down. Test the temperature with your forearm. If the heat is bearable, then prepare to sit down over the steam.

- Place a small pillow behind your back for comfort. Sit down on the toilet seat.

- Open your legs and cover your body from the waist down with a large towel to trap the steam.

- Quiet your mind and close your eyes. Do deep breathing exercises. Sit and relax for 30 minutes.

<u>**Padsicles**</u>

After a vaginal birth, that area may be sore. It has been stretched enormously and probably even torn or cut (episiotomy) during delivery. Stitches may have been required to repair the perineum and/or even the anus. Whatever the outcome is, after vaginal childbirth the labia, vaginal opening, perineum and anal region deserves some special attention. Use padsicles often to relieve any vaginal discomfort. These pads may offer healing to the delicate skin tissues.

How to make Padsicles

<u>Materials</u>
7 Menstrual Pads
Aloe Vera Gel
Herbs *(calendula, rose, lavender)*
Water
Pot (2 Quarts)

<u>Instructions</u>

- Make an herbal infusion by adding 1 cup of herbs to a pot filled with 1 quart of boiling water.

- Cover with a lid and remove from the heating source. Allow it to cool down, then use the herbal infusion after a few hours.

- Open the menstrual pad and pour about ¼ cup of the herbal infusion inside.

- Add ¼ cup of aloe vera gel into the menstrual pads.

- Fold the pad inward, seal with wrapper and store in the freezer till frozen.

Belly Binding

During pregnancy, your body grows and stretches to accommodate your baby. To make space, your abdominal muscles separate, and organs move out of their normal position.

Belly binding is an ancient cultural tradition of wrapping the hips, belly, and torso of postpartum women tightly with a long piece of non-stretch fabric. This practice offers abdominal support, stability, and comfort to the muscles, skin, and internal organs to repair and bring healing to the postpartum body.

Childbirth can take a toll on the body and the uterus needs to shrink back to its original size. There is also emotional healing provided to the postpartum mother. It can ease muscle tension and give a soothing, closing up feeling. Binding is an excellent way to heal the muscle walls back together and also support the spine and posture realignment. It can assist in the healing process of the uterus. Wrapping the belly can help your belly return to its pre-pregnancy size. It is best to be done on the naked body. Remove clothing before you begin. Binding should feel secure and supportive but not uncomfortable and should definitely not interfere with breathing. Wait at least an hour after eating before you belly bind.

When done properly, belly binding applied to the abdomen and around the hips can provide support to your pelvic floor. It also offers gentle compression that holds muscle and ligaments safely in place as your body heals.

Belly binding is meant to gently hold your mid-section in place, supporting your core and encouraging your body to heal. Be careful not to wrap it too tightly as this can be problematic to your health. You should not be struggling to breathe or unable to function as you normally would. It's normal to feel some compression, but not to the point that you can't move.

Wear for up to 18 hours per day, but not while sleeping for a few months after childbirth. You will need several yards of fabric (about 14–18 yards), preferably muslin. Your doula, partner, family member or friend can help you bind your belly. This is not something that you can do alone.

You can start from day 1 after birth and continue for 40+ days. It doesn't matter what type of birth you've had (vaginal or cesarean), you can receive the benefits.

<u>Belly Bind Instructions</u>

- Wrap the fabric comfortably and completely around the belly without any clothing underneath, directly against the skin.
- Tighten the wrap just enough to feel compression, but not tightness. The wrap should always remain comfortable to wear.
- Remove the wrap before going to bed.

<u>Postpartum Depression</u>

After a woman delivers a baby, she may struggle with hopelessness and sadness. She could be happy one minute, then in full-blown tears the next. Fortunately, these depressive feelings and thoughts typically go away within weeks of delivery for some women. Observe any mood changes, anxiety and crying after childbirth. These symptoms could become more persistent or severe, which could indicate postpartum depression. If you have the desire to hurt yourself or your baby, seek help immediately.

Childbirth is a life-changing event and can bring on a myriad of emotions. A woman has literally created and grown another human and now has the responsibility of caring for them. When a woman is cared for, just as delicately as the baby, the rate of depression can be greatly reduced.

<u>**15 Ways to Prevent Postpartum Depression**</u>

1. Write down your feelings in your ***Pregnancy Journal***.
2. Speak 5 affirmations aloud to yourself 3 times per day.
3. Spend some time outdoors.
4. Allow sunlight into your home.
5. Go for a swim.
6. Take a candlelit bath.
7. Go for a walk.
8. Meditate/Pray, do your spiritual preference daily.
9. Eat nutritious meals and drink herbal tea.
10. Be around positive people who want the best for you.
11. Leave your child(ren) with someone whom you trust and enjoy a break.
12. Practice a hobby. Do something creative with your mind or hands.
13. Talk to a professional therapist.
14. Talk to a trusted friend; have a good conversation.
15. Watch a funny movie or television show.

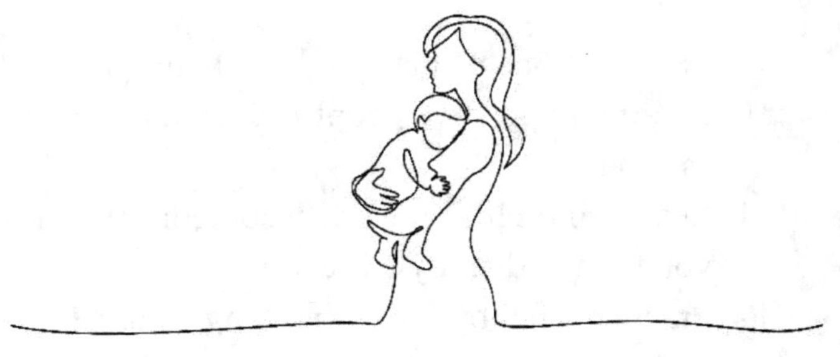

Abena Adu | 64

Conclusion

My intent is that you will look at bringing in life through a different lens. By applying the knowledge in this book, you now have the capability of changing the path of maternal and infant mortality. Complications can also decrease with being consistently proactive in reaching health goals. It all starts with education. We must know better in order to do better.

Mate selection, preparing the body and intentionally conceiving is the foundation. Being assertive, physically active, and eating healthy is a great median. End with a satisfying delivery and postpartum experience.

No matter what the current statistics are, we all should unify in the effort to create better pregnancy, birth and postpartum outcomes.

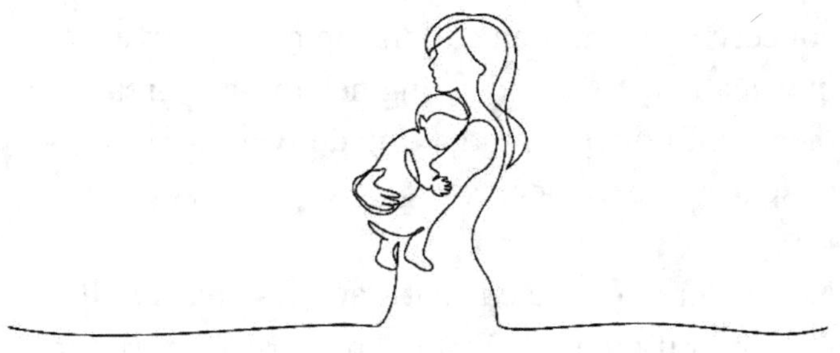

About the Author

Abena Adu is an author, educator, certified doula and midwife assistant. She has experienced a medicated hospital birth and unassisted home births. She defied the odds and successfully birthed healthy children in her so-called "advanced maternal age," all while also being labeled "high risk."

Abena enjoys helping women with womb healing, fertility, home birthing and lactation. She offers courses and consultations. You may find her teaching a class near you.

Abena is a proud wife and mother who enjoys preparing vegan food and traveling.

Other Books by this Author

The Dark Womb Redemption: A Holistic Guide to Womb Wellness for Black Women

The Dark Womb Redemption Workbook

The Dark Womb Redemption 3: A Guide to Fertility, Homebirth and Breastfeeding

Pregnancy Journal

www.ingramcontent.com/pod-product-compliance
Lightning Source LLC
Chambersburg PA
CBHW061306250726
48653CB00002B/807